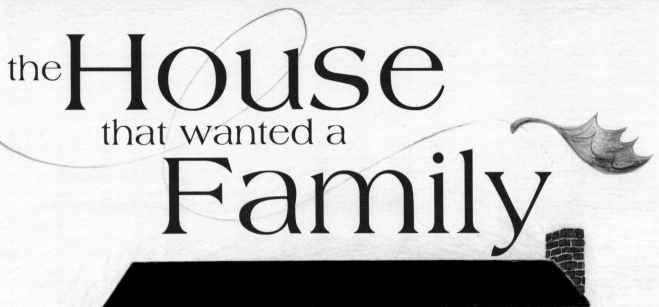

the House that wanted a Family

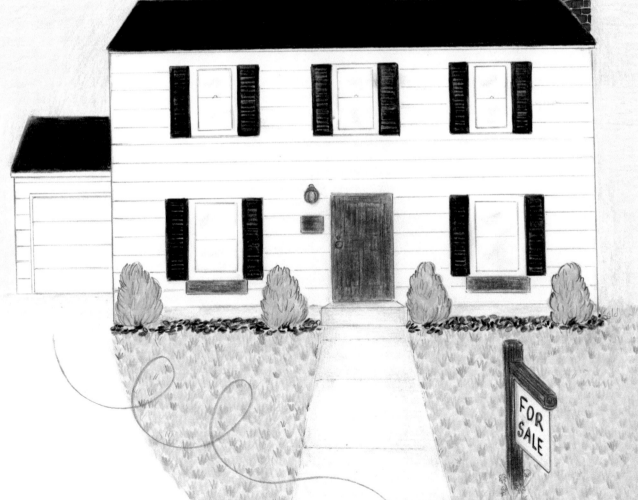

Susan Spence Daniel

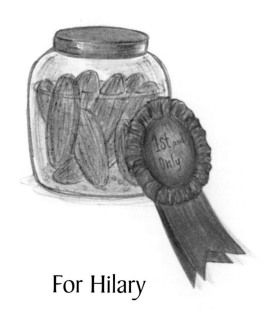

For Hilary

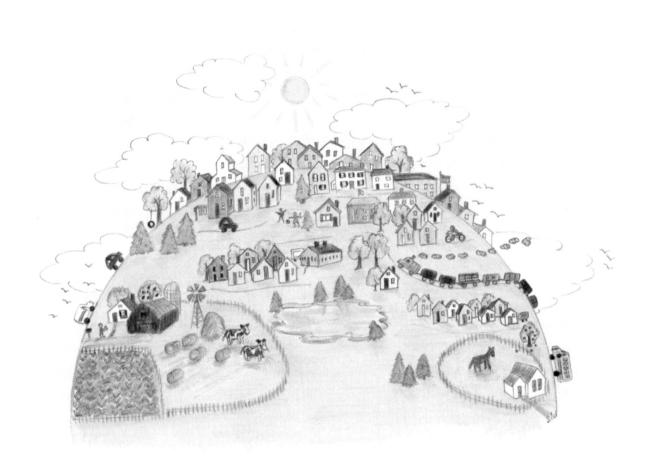

In a town, not too big and not too small, there was a house.

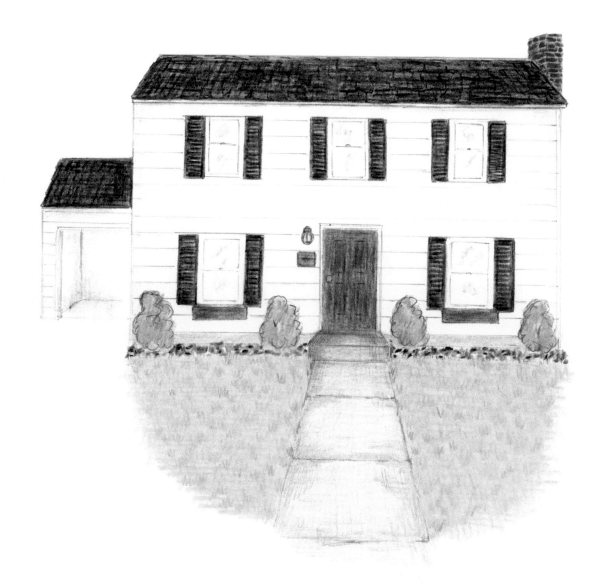

The house was like the other houses on the street except for one thing: it was empty. There was no furniture in the rooms and there were no clothes in the closets. There were no books on the bookshelves or dishes in the cupboards. And there was no car in the garage.

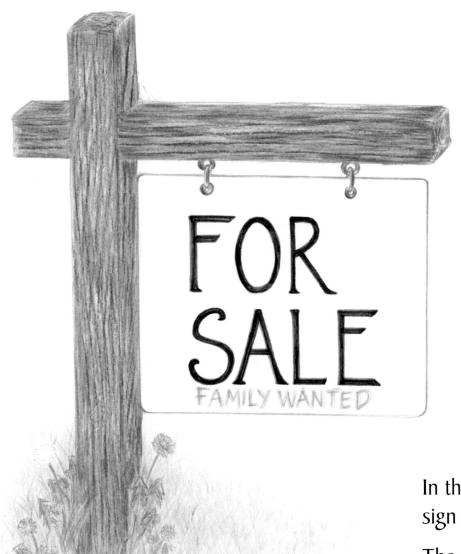

In the front yard was a large sign that read "FOR SALE."

The sign had been there a long time.

The house thought the sign should say "Family Wanted."

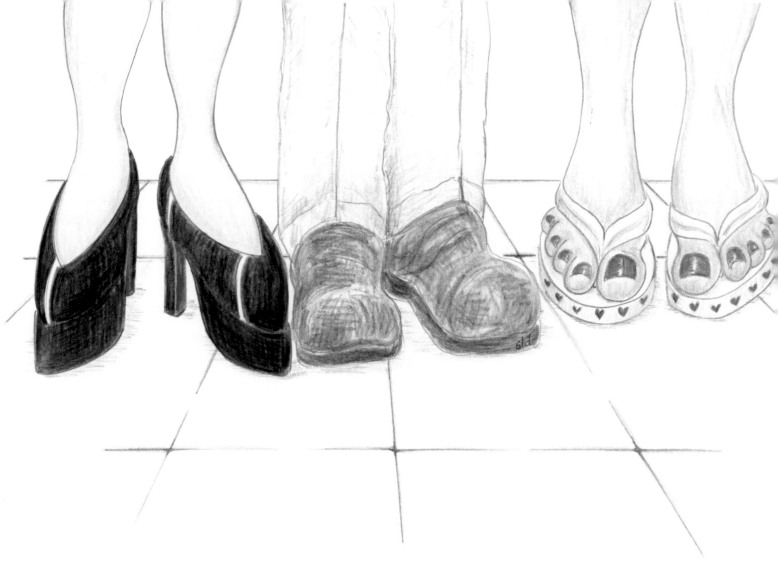

Sometimes people came and walked around the yard and through the house. Some of the people spoke quietly to each other, and some of the people talked rather loudly.

A lady wearing very tall
shoes and fancy pearls
announced that there
weren't enough closets.

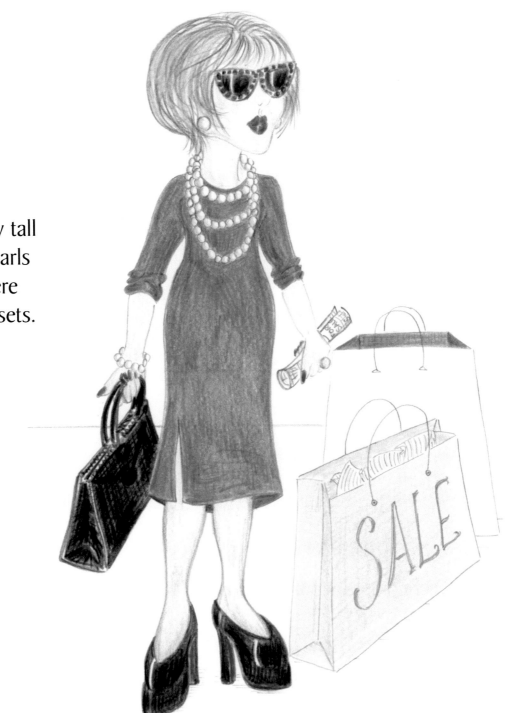

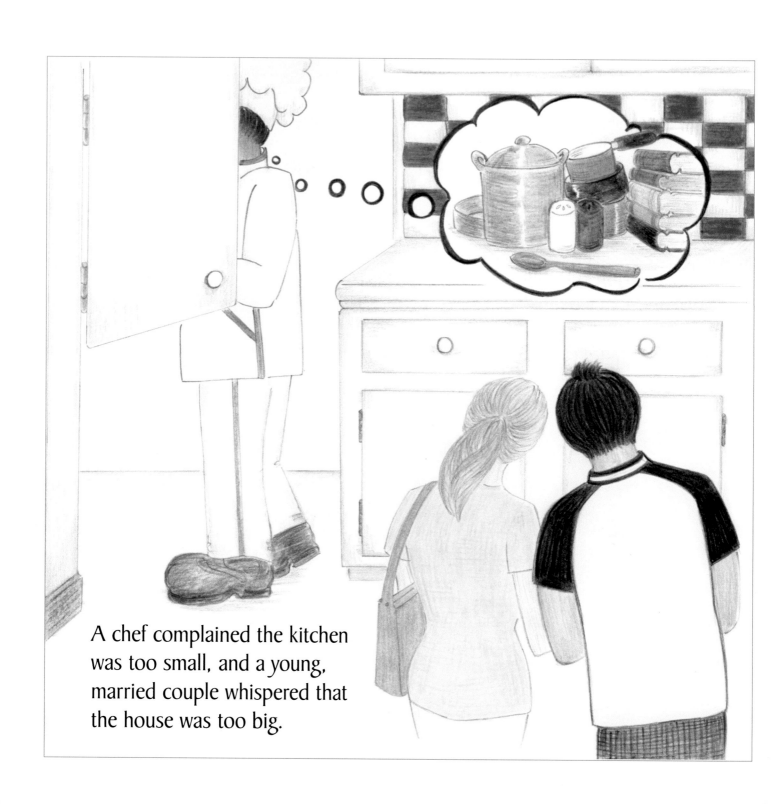

A chef complained the kitchen was too small, and a young, married couple whispered that the house was too big.

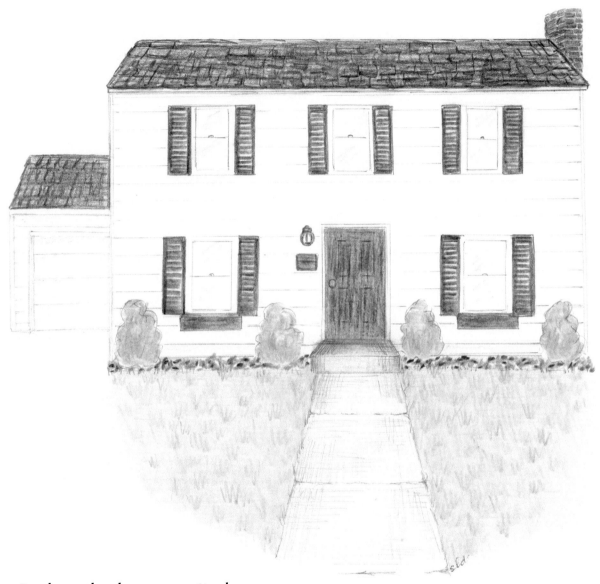

And so the house waited.

And it waited.

And it waited.

In the beginning, the windows were clean, the lawn was neat and tidy, and the house looked ready for company.

But that was in the beginning.

Over time, things started to change.

The windows became dusty and dirty. Leaves and pieces of paper rolled and tumbled in the yard. Some of them became caught in the bushes and stayed there for several days or weeks.

The house began to look sad and neglected.

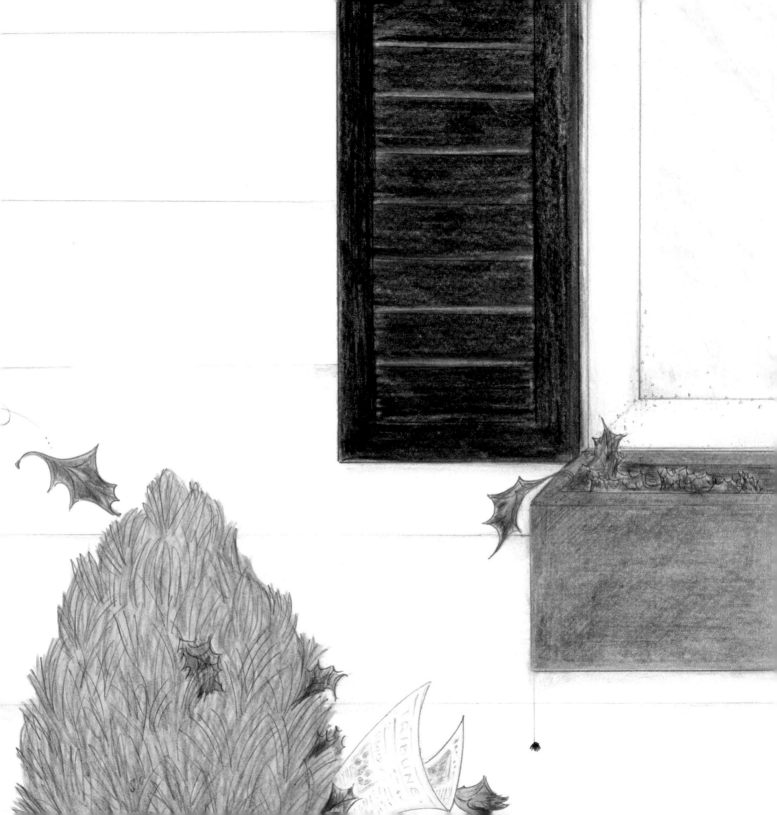

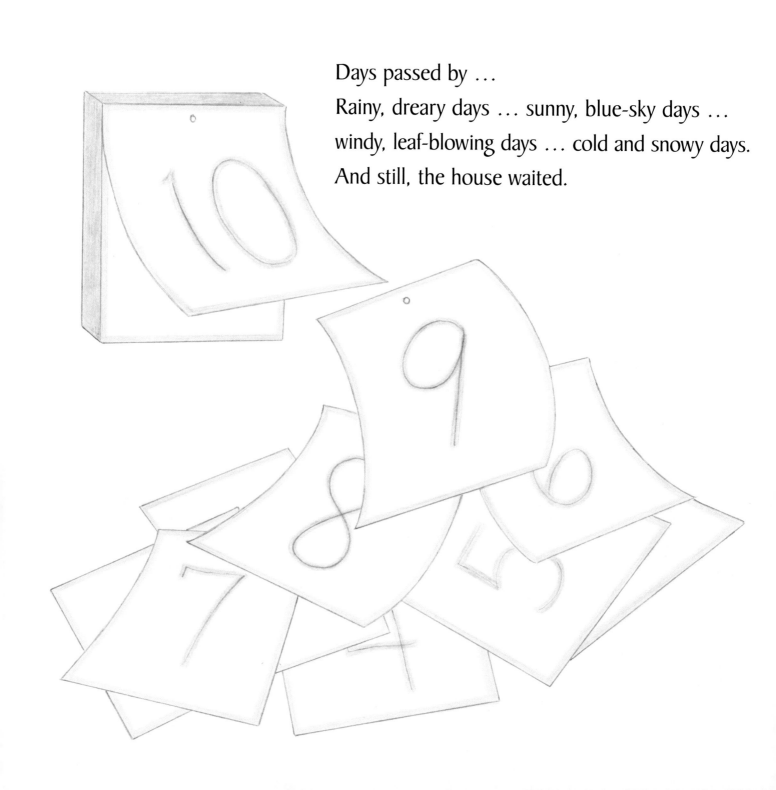

Days passed by ...
Rainy, dreary days ... sunny, blue-sky days ...
windy, leaf-blowing days ... cold and snowy days.
And still, the house waited.

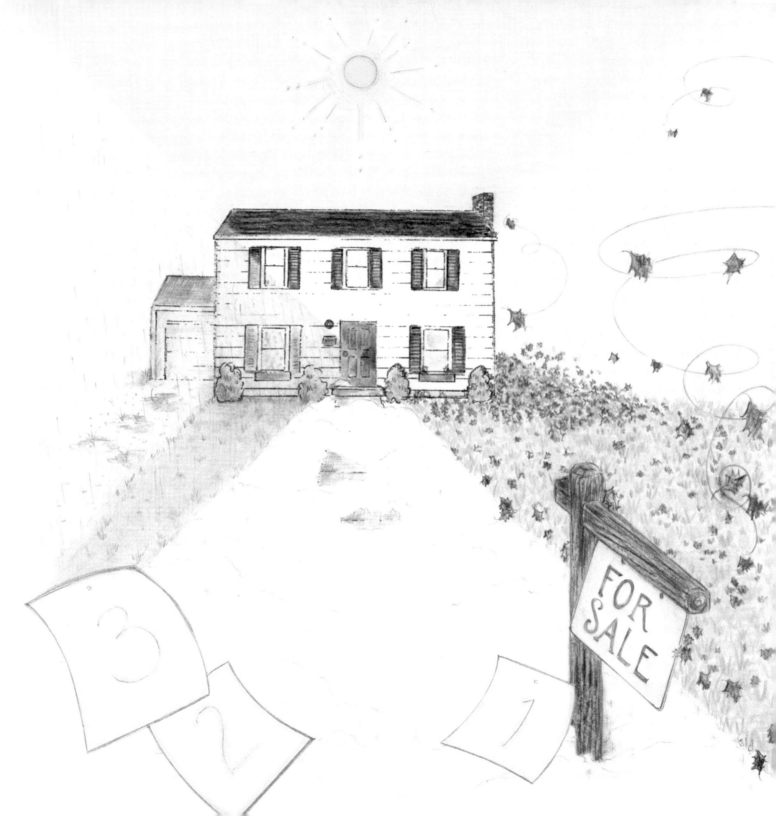

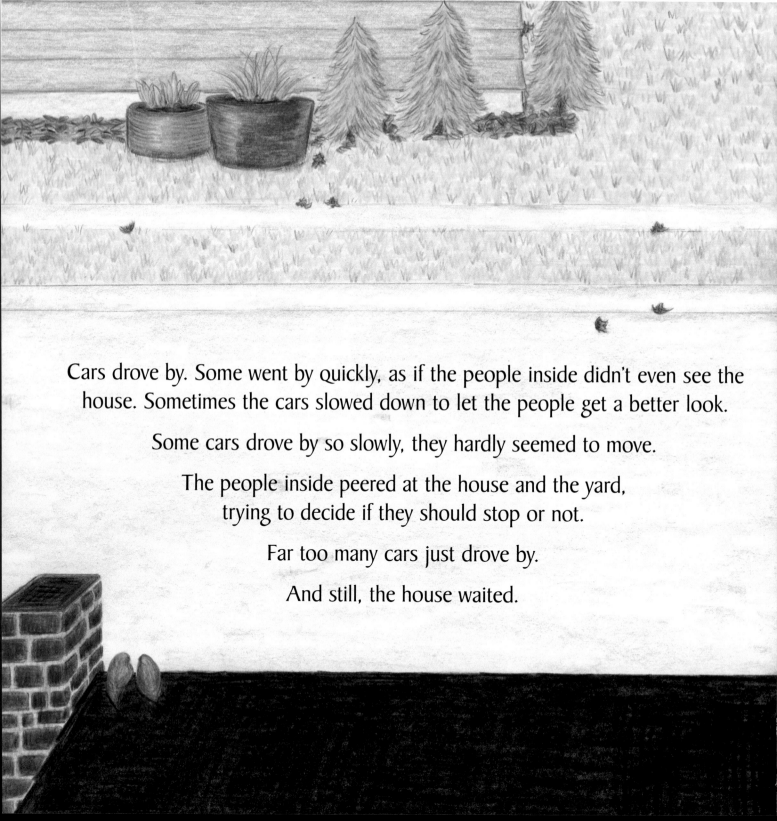

Cars drove by. Some went by quickly, as if the people inside didn't even see the house. Sometimes the cars slowed down to let the people get a better look.

Some cars drove by so slowly, they hardly seemed to move.

The people inside peered at the house and the yard,
trying to decide if they should stop or not.

Far too many cars just drove by.

And still, the house waited.

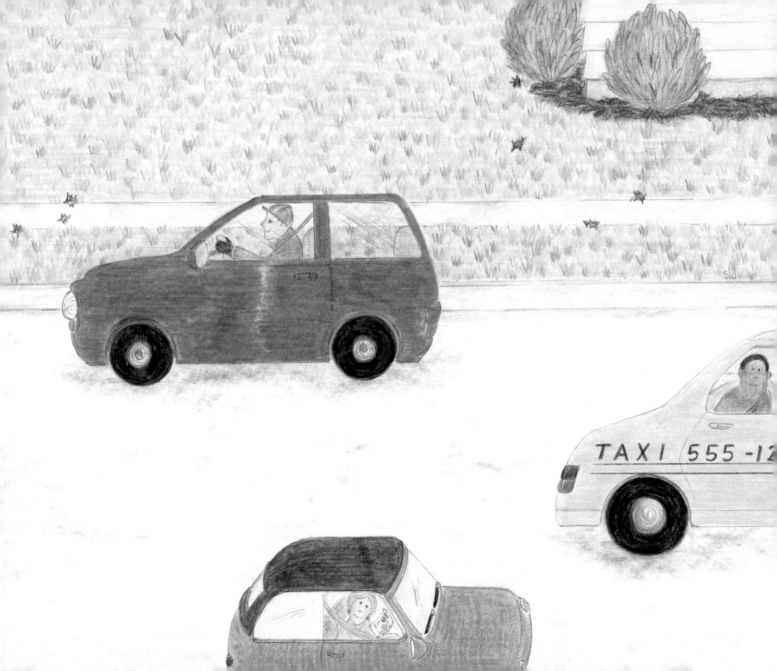

Then, one day, a van drove by … stopped …
backed up … and pulled into the driveway.
And one after another, the doors opened and out came …

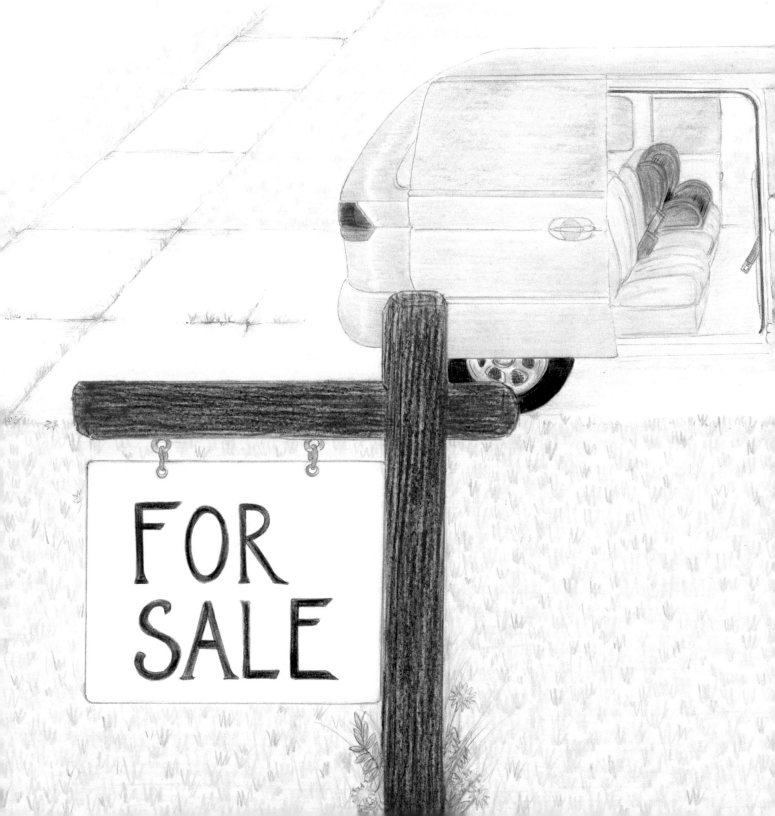

A family!

The house could hardly contain itself.

As the family walked around the yard and into the house, they exclaimed together,

"This is just what we've been looking for!"

The house smiled.

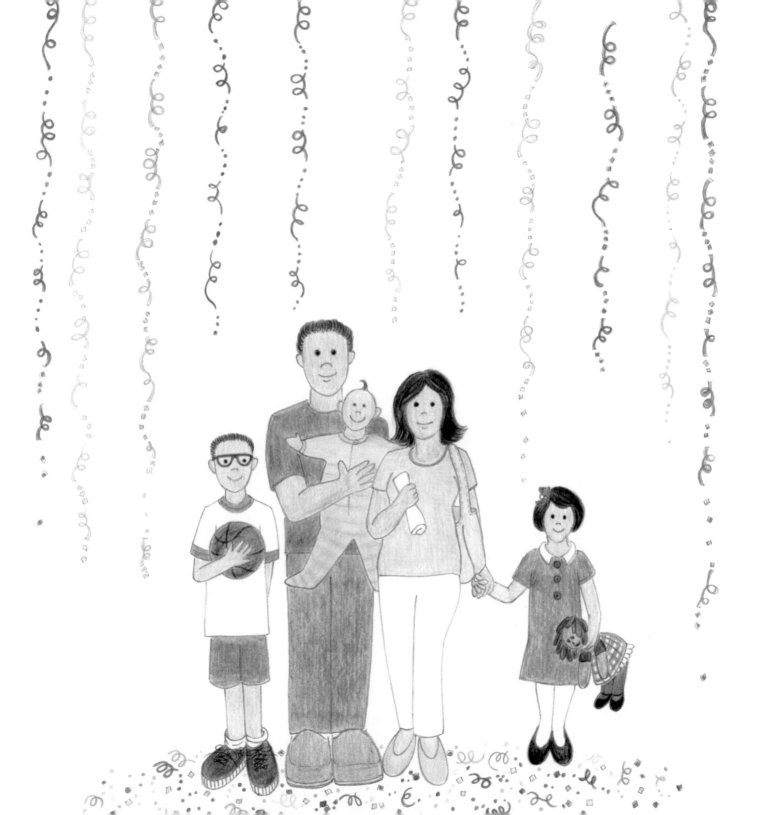

Before too many more days and nights went by, a big truck pulled up to the house and backed into the driveway.

Out of the truck came boxes and furniture and toys.

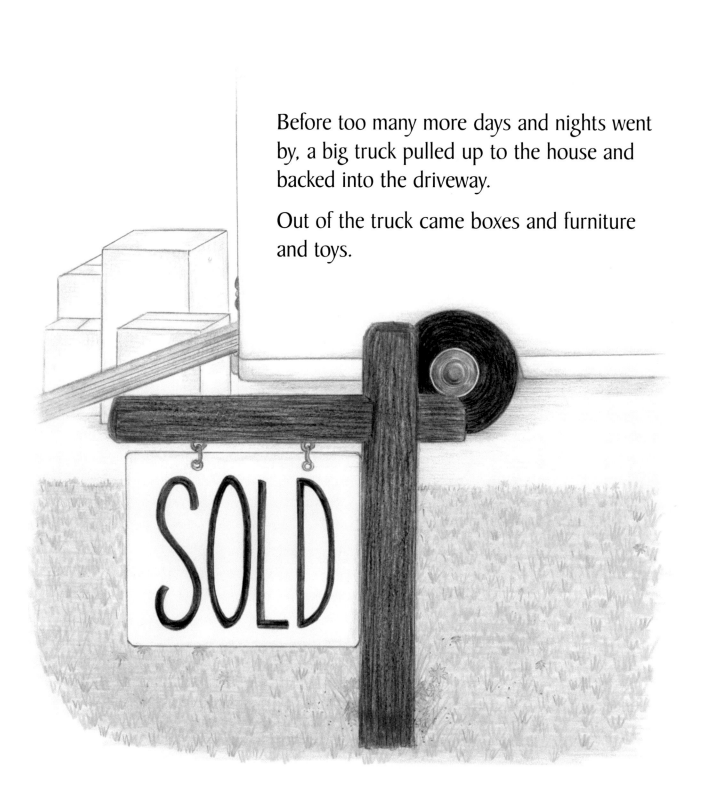

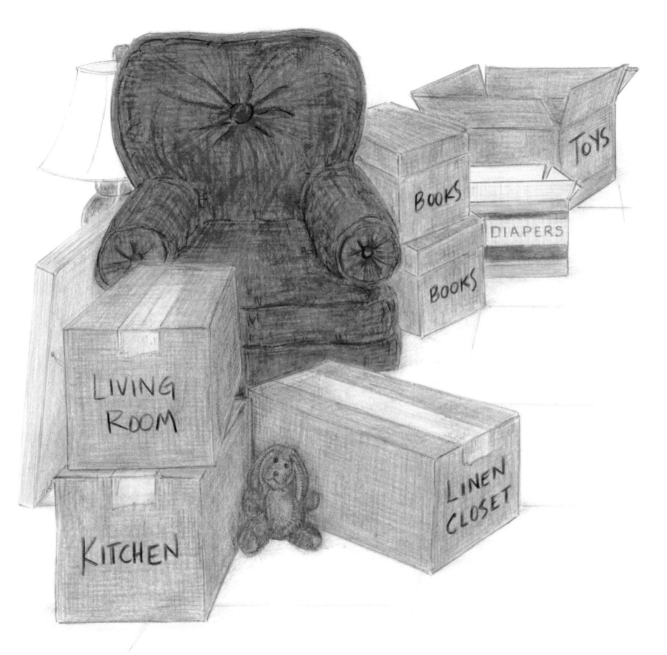

The family filled the rooms with their things.

But mostly they filled the house with their love.

Inviting smells soon made their way throughout the house—coffee brewing, cookies baking, and the smoky smell of logs and pinecones burning in the fireplace.

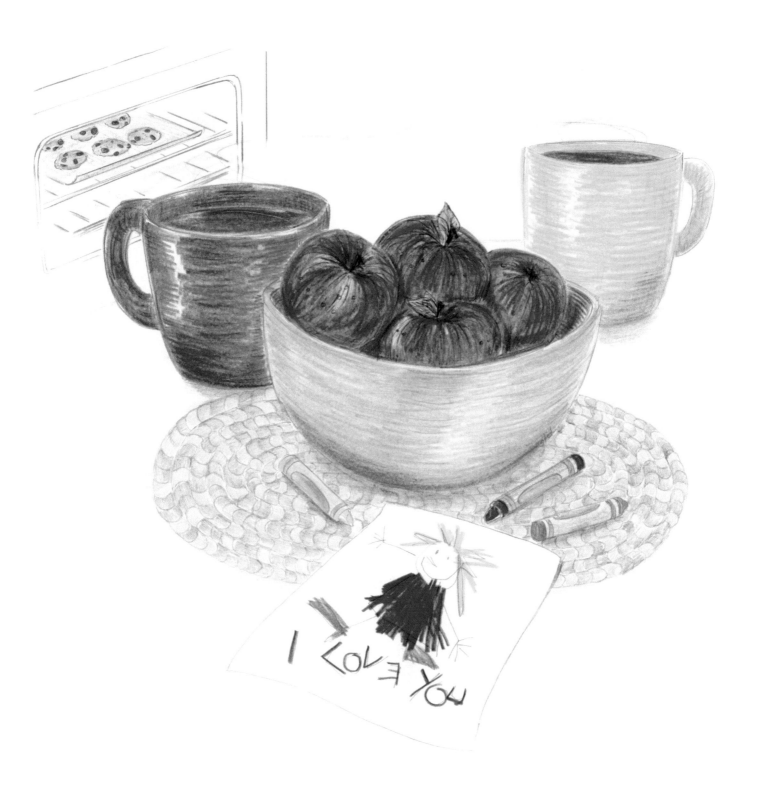

Sometimes smells from outside found their way into the house: clothes drying on the clothesline, freshly cut grass, and food sizzling on the grill.

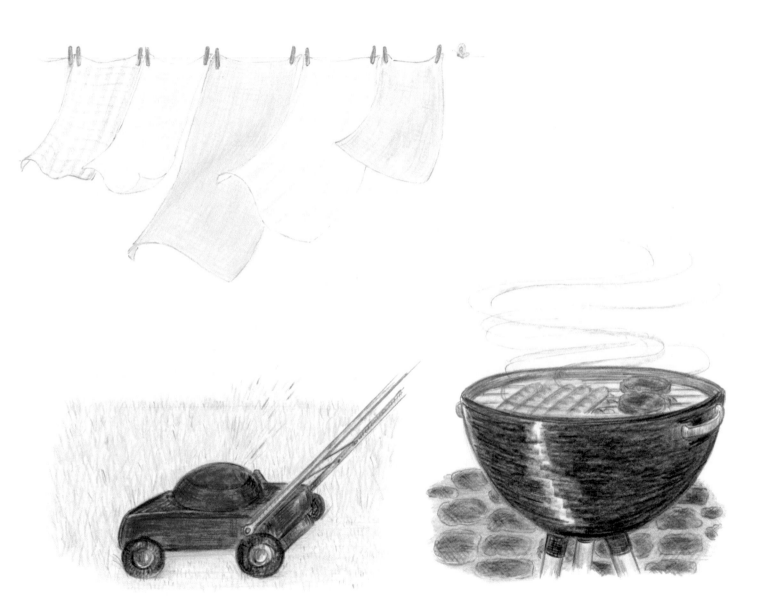

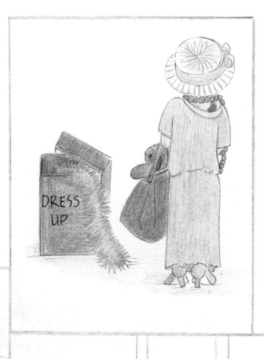

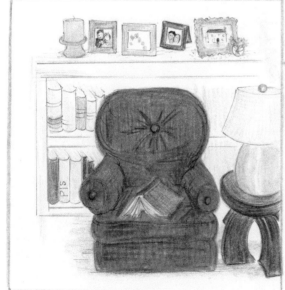

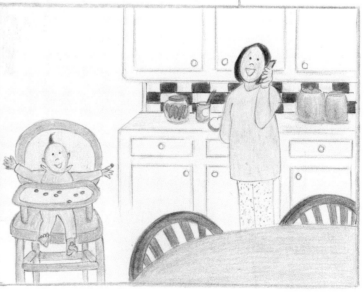

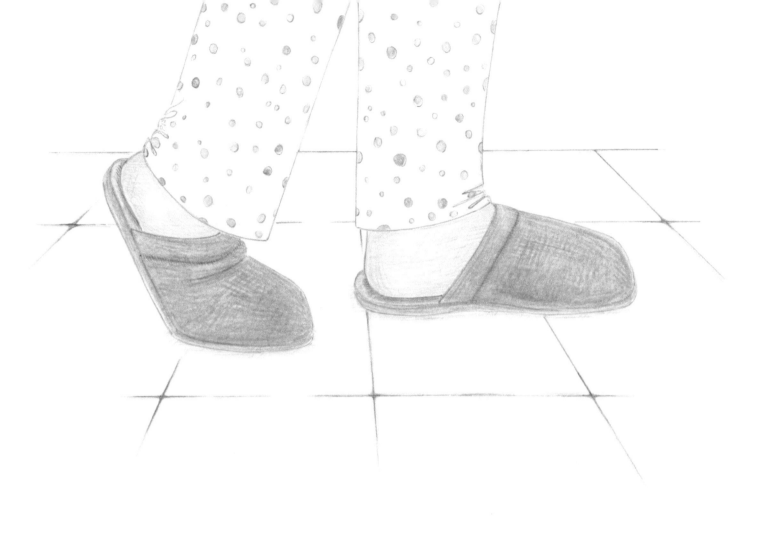

No longer quiet, the rooms echoed with the sounds of a family: voices and laughter, singing and music, running feet and slippered shuffles that tickled the floors and the ears of all who heard them.

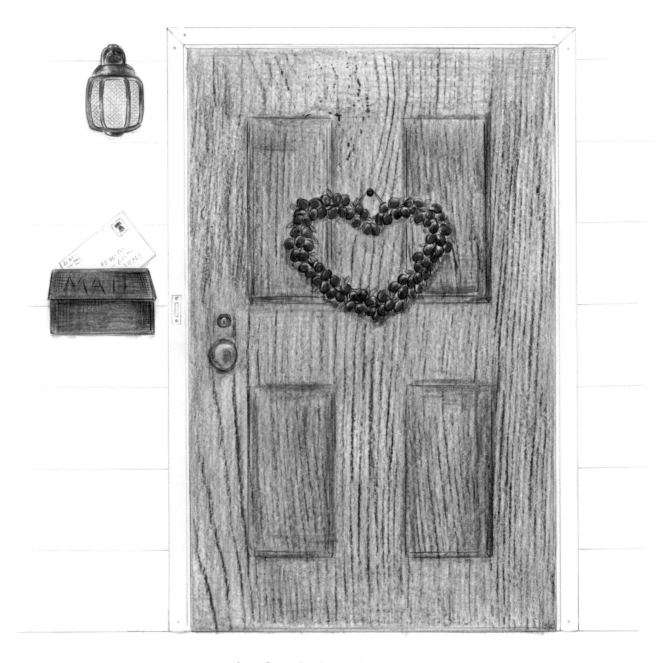

The family loved the house.
And the house loved them back.

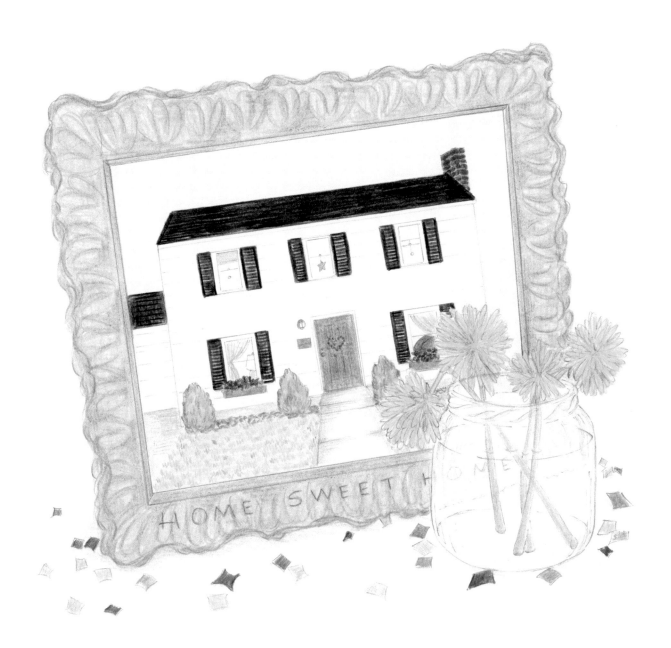

And then, the most wonderful thing happened.
The house that had waited so long for a family … became a home.

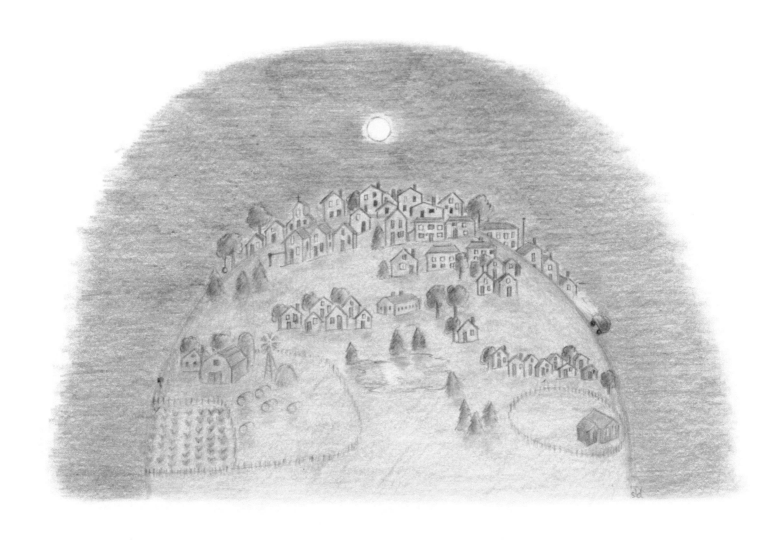

Inspiring Voices books may be ordered through booksellers or by contacting:

Inspiring Voices
1663 Liberty Drive
Bloomington, IN 47403
www.inspiringvoices.com
1 (844) 686-9605

Layout Assistance: Laurie Liebewein Spence
Author Photo: Joan Richio
The illustrations in this book were done in pencil color with pencil outline.

ISBN: 978-1-4624-0081-2 (sc)
ISBN: 978-1-4624-0167-3 (e)

Library of Congress Control Number: 2012934596

Print information available on the last page.

Inspiring Voices rev. date: 03/02/2021

InspiringVoices®